THE CAREGIVER OF THE ACTIVE PATIENT

7 Aspects That Affected Me

ISABEL WALBOURNE

IngramSpark: Self-Publishing Book Company, Inc.
http://www.ingramspark.com

ISBN: 978-1-64945-630-4 – Paperback
ISBN: 978-1-64945-632-8 – cBook

To my family and friends that have
been through this.
And to all Caregivers that need this.

Table of Contents:

   A. Learn about the illness your loved one is going through.
   B. Physical reactions to the drugs taken.
   C. Physical appearance and long-term use of the drugs.
   D. Food and plastic tableware.
   E. Physical activity.

   A. At the doctors, when the wall comes down.
   B. The world of pain is only their arm's length.
   C. Change of personality.
   D. Why me?
   E. I can still drive the car!
   F. Don't give me that stuff! I don't want it! I want to go home!
   G. Talk about plans for the future.
   H. Talk to the children.

Foreword

There was a lot of pain involved with going through cancer and surgeries. Besides painful, it was frustrating to no end: there was a lot of crying by myself, no one seemed to know what it was like, and I didn't want anyone to see me until I was healthy again. I just didn't know it would take a year and a half to get to remission, nor that it would take another few years to get healthy again. Well, as healthy as I was going to get.

My body seemed to be in pain all the time. Eating and drinking fluids interrupted what little rest I could get. It was mostly by exhaustion that I would finally fall asleep, and then it was time to get up and walk the block. Or eat something only to throw it up. Or go to an appointment at the doctor's or the hospital to be poked with needles, prodded with scopes, and lie uncomfortably on tables for x-rays. For a year and a half, I was in this constant state. How can you blame me for being "grumpy"? I was not a monster—I was in *pain!*

Chemotherapy, in my day, was the shotgun effect. The chemicals were shot into my veins, and we hoped the bad cells would get eliminated without too many of the good cells being killed off as well. The progression of technology has gotten to where two lasers can do a better job of eliminating a bad cell without touching a good cell. I wish they had been able to do that during my turn with cancer.

That being said, I would never have survived without my wife pushing me to do all this. I would have given up by the second surgery. I didn't want any more surgeries. I just wanted to lay down and die so the pain would stop.

There are leftover effects that remain to this day: surgical staples that held my intestines in the right place, so naturally, I set off airport metal detectors and have to show them the long scar. I lost half my lungs to the chemicals and had to train them to expand so I could breathe normally. And I have tinnitus. Hearing aids also puts volume to the tinnitus and is just as hard to hear everything else around it.

As anyone who has gone through a fight with cancer will tell you, I did not beat it. I survived it. But only with the help of a pushy caregiver, my wife.

Gary Walbourne, the Impatient Patient

Introduction

There are plenty of papers, pamphlets, and books to help a caregiver with information. From the doctors and nurses to the library and "Google-ing", the methods for caring for any disabled person to a bed-ridden invalid seem to have no limit. But not much information is readily available for taking care of the active patient or the caregiver. Although many have taken care of an ill person in their family, one becomes a caregiver when a loved one becomes ill with a long-term illness, disease, disability, or death of another loved one. Not only does the ill person need be to taken care of, but so does the rest of the family. And so do you, the caregiver.

Please be assured, I am not a nurse. I am not a doctor. I am not a pharmacist. I am not a person of specialized training. I am simply a daughter, a wife, and a working mother. With the law of averages, it takes two of our incomes to pay for and keep our house. As my husband owned his own business, it was my health insurance from my job that helped pay for large portions of the doctor bills, hospital bills, and pharmacies. At one point, I had 24 invoices of separate visits to the hospital in one year. Try keeping that straight!

After dealing with my husband's week-long near spinal meningitis and year-and-a-half cancer fight, my role as a caregiver became very informative for others that began to have similar experiences. All the people's names in this small booklet, except for doctors, if mentioned, are fictional to protect their privacy. I have tried to keep all names out so that this booklet could be meant for anyone and everyone that must care for a family member or ill person. What I am trying to describe is what might work for more than just what worked for my family. I am hoping this will inform people that there are other standards that can be used for you, the caregiver, with a patient that is still up on their feet and driving you crazy.

It seems the categories of the physical illness, the mindset of your loved one, the psychological and spiritual beliefs, and the social offset by the loved one shunning the outside world, is all from a mind of the ill person that is still cognizant of what is going on. Not only are you, the caregiver, having to deal with all this, but this loved one you would love to strangle is running circles around your mind, as well as the house, the hospital, and/or the workplace, if they are lucky to keep their job. In my instance, with my husband's business, there was no question about not going back to work.

There is no set order in reading this booklet. Please go to whatever section is needed for the moment. You can always go back to another subject later. Or you can read it at your leisure when you have some spare time. (Spare time? What is that?)

Chapter 1 – The Physical Aspect
A. Learn about the illness your loved one is going through.

I did not know it at the time, but Gary, my husband, initiated my care-giving training when he was struck by a cold gone wild. We were living with Gary's mother, along with our two boys, then 3 and 7 years old. Gary had a head cold around Thanksgiving time, fighting off the blocked sinuses and a sore throat. We were Christmas shopping on the first day of December, stopping for lunch at a restaurant. As we sat waiting for our food to arrive, Gary's face color became pale and grayish. So instead of continuing our shopping, we decided to go home so he could get some rest.

Lying on the sofa, Gary began shaking from being cold. He had a fever, and his shaking began to vibrate the sofa so hard that the window curtains also shook. I woke him up and told him to get to bed. He moved to go to the bedroom, but then had to go to the bathroom to throw up.

After getting him into bed and setting up a bagged trash can to throw up in, Gary tried to sleep. He was restless, complaining I should have left him alone, swinging his arms from one side to the other, and after every three times, he would miss the trash can. It was when he incoherently asked for something to drink that I called his doctor.

By now, Gary was finally getting a little bit of rest, but it seemed every fifteen minutes to a half hour, he was up again and reaching for the trash can. I couldn't get him to drink water as that would set him off to throwing up again. It got so bad that when he sat up, he looked at the trash can, looked the other way, and threw up on the bed next to himself. I thought I couldn't handle it. Then he lay back down and put his arm through it and under the pillow.

As it happened, the doctor was going to leave for his vacation on this Saturday afternoon. It took three hours to get a call back from him, and he told me to take Gary to the

Emergency Room to get him to stop vomiting. He would dehydrate very quickly and end up there anyway.

Pulling off Gary's dirty T-shirt was easy compared to Mom and me trying to get a clean one on. It was like wrestling with a 200-pound gorilla to put his arms into the holes of the shirt. He called me every family name of authority, but mine. I suppose I didn't represent any authority over him. With Mom's help, we finally managed it and had him dressed in sweatpants and slippers, too. Getting him outside to the car with both of us at his side, the cold night air hit him, and he had to take a whiz—in the bushes. We didn't want to take the chance of losing the ground we had gained by leading him back into the house.

With trash can in his hands, I left Mom to stay home with the boys. I had to circle for a landing at getting to the hospital Emergency Room, as it was also the time of the Christmas parade. Finally, I had Gary wait in the car and went into the Emergency Room to get paperwork started. I asked for a wheelchair so I would not have to help Gary walk in. I told the nurse that he was throwing up, and she handed me a little ear cleaning dish, as that was all she had. Uh-uh. The trash can came with Gary into the room.

Maybe an hour later, a doctor finally came to see Gary. Giving the history of his head cold, sore throat, and ear infection, the doctor told us he will have to do a spinal tap. I let him know he would need two strong interns to hold Gary down, or he would not be successful. I could hear Gary cry out as I was walking down the hall. My father-in-law was walking to me, also hearing Gary, and we stayed together in the waiting room. We found out later that Gary had struck the doctor, as the nurse that was holding him failed to keep him subdued. It took another hour or two to get a hospital room before I could go home.

At 2:30 a.m., I arrived home, unable to go to sleep, because there was this mess on the bed. I had to remove the covers and sheets, start them in the washing machine, wash the mattress, wash the bedroom carpet spots, put towels down to keep from getting too wet, and put new sheets and blanket on. I finally fell asleep about 3:45 a.m. At 6 a.m., one kid had to be up and going to school, the other to go with Grandma to the shop. I finally got to the hospital again at about 7:30 a.m.

Gary was awake and complaining about his T-shirt smelling like puke. Well, it was a clean shirt going onto a dirty body. I gave him a sponge bath and he changed into another clean shirt I had brought in for him. It wasn't until we got to talk to the doctors that we could ask about what was happening.

We learned that spinal meningitis was striking down several people very seriously that year. My father-in-law had an employee's son of 23 years old who had a headache, was dehydrated, and went to the hospital. He died within three days. Dad was scared it was happening to his 33-year-old son. Gary ended up staying four days in the hospital, getting 400,000 units of penicillin a day. There's no pill big enough for that much dosage.

But what confused me was how Gary almost got this spinal meningitis. What was it? Why did it suddenly get so bad? Where did it come from? These are the questions I asked the doctors.

The answers were logical but astounding to me. Because Gary's cold had been with him for several weeks, from his throat and sinuses to his ear infection, his doctor had put him on a cough suppressant that had codeine in it. Gary really did not normally get sick. He was always healthy as a horse! When the allergic reaction to the codeine began making Gary throw up, the infection decided to go elsewhere. From the ears, the spinal cord and brain are the closest areas of where to move. When Gary could not raise his chin very high, the doctor said it might be the spinal meningitis threat. The spinal tap was to see if any infection had gone into the spinal cord to the brain. Thankfully, it had not, but the doctor was not very good at doing the spinal tap and hit bone, which is very painful, so he got hit for it.

This was my initiation into care giving.

When Gary got sick again a year or so later it was just a stomachache that he couldn't get rid of. He did not feel like eating because he felt like he was constipated or something. It did not go away in a day or two, and he had to sit up to feel like he could go to sleep. After three days, I suggested he go to the doctor. No, no, it's just a stomachache. It took another sleepless night sitting on the sofa for him to decide to go see the doctor.

After the first examination, the General Practice doctor suggested that it might very well be his stomach ulcer acting up. Pain pills for aches, change his diet with eating soft foods, and no spices were listed. A week later, the pain was worse, the diet did not seem to help, and the doctor gave him stronger pain pills. Another week and Gary and I decided that if there was no change of prescribing what to do, we would go find another doctor to talk to.

Well, the doctor was a step ahead of us. He had asked another doctor and a surgeon what might be causing this stomach pain. There might be a better way of finding out what was going on inside with a scope. The esophagus gastroscopy was done. That's a camera tube going down the throat to see what's going on in the stomach. They found the old ulcer, which was not flared up, and tried going into the small intestine. It seemed to be stuck after a short way. Next, the Barium Enema for the Lower GI (gastro-intestinal), which did not show anything either; and the tube got stuck halfway up the large intestine, as well.

We at least thought this was some progress in finding out what was going on with Gary's body. As there was nothing to be seen on the inside of the organs, the doctors thought there might be something on the outside of the organs. An MRI was scheduled for the next week, which was on a Friday. Gary remembers the nurse gasping at what she saw as she took the images. The MRI was done at 9 a.m. We got a call at 11:30 a.m. We had an Oncology appointment at 3 p.m.

This was the beginning of a year and a half of taking care of my husband, my kids, keeping at my job, and doing more things than I ever thought possible, because I simply had to do it all. There was no one else to do it for me. Many people I have talked to feel like they can't do any more.

I let them know that they *can* do it, and they *will* do it, simply because they *have* to do it.

The next week, Gary was set up for an exploratory surgery. Afterwards, I was numb with shock for the few minutes the doctor was telling me about it. They could not find the source of the tumor of where it came from, could not take out the tumor for the tendrils going around his organs, and could not tell what kind of tumor it was. He was afraid of hitting even a capillary where the cancer cells would spread like wildfire. Gary would be dead in two weeks if it got into his bloodstream. I stared at him in disbelief. When he was done explaining this to me and left, I turned to my mother who was sitting with me and burst into tears.

What could I do? How did Gary get a tumor? Why did he get this thing? And how do I tell my husband they left the tumor inside him? How long before the doctors would know from the tests they began of what kind of cancer it is? How do we fight this thing? How long does he have to live if it doesn't go away? And what do I do if Gary dies and I am left with two small children, then aged 5 and 9, to raise on my own? I wouldn't know what to do with his company, the equipment in the shop, and his mother and I with no income from it. My resolve was that I could not let him die on me.

I was a Data Entry clerk at a medical clinic with 32 doctors, working from 5 p.m. to 11 p.m. This way, by not working regular day hours, we did not have to have a babysitter. I keyed in office visits, laboratory tests, x-rays, and diagnosis codes, as well as the hospital visit charges that all the doctors did in their hospital rounds. I spent the next year and a half keying in all of Gary's charges as they were happening. It frightened me to see the $50,000 and more at a time going into his records, relief that the insurance covered much of it, and discouraged to put more charges in again. Some of my work breaks were spent in a quiet place where I could just sit and stare out into the night, hoping I wouldn't break down too often in front of my coworkers.

The clinic was lucky to have Dr. Miguel Garcia, Surgeon and Urologist, who rated 3rd in the state of California at the time. He immediately saw that the cancer was from a testicular tumor that had escaped into the open cavity outside of the organs. Gary's body had already destroyed the testicle that had started it, but there were too many damaged cells for his body to get it all. A quick surgery took it out. Now this kind of testicular cancer is commonly known as the Lance Armstrong disease. If it is caught early enough, there is a 99% chance of success in getting rid of it. Had Gary's cancer not escaped into his body cavity, it might have been detected sooner.

By the next week with his scheduled Chemotherapy, one of his kidneys was shut off, the other one half closed, and two strong tendrils were wrapping around his heart. A small lump on his neck started that morning. That is a swelling lymph node giving a sign that the cancer is spreading to more than just the organs.

Dr. Sharon Yee, Gary's Oncologist, said that usually this is the first sign that anyone notices they have a lump. And they think, "Oh, it will go away." A month later when they come to see a doctor, it is already too late. Dr Yee revels in the fact that Gary survived, as 80% of her patients die. After three surgeries with Dr. Yee inside and outside of his body, she was on a first-name basis with Gary.

Learning about this particular cancer gave us a small hope that Gary would live if he can survive the Chemotherapy and added surgery to remove the tumor. It had been proven there was a 95% success rate with this combination of cancer fighting. I told Dr. Yee to get started.

When an illness or a disease strikes learn about it so you can find out how to fight it.

Testicular cancer is known as the White Man's disease. It normally strikes men of Caucasian European decent, mostly between the ages of 18 to 35 years of age. Medically speaking, each race may have its own peculiar idiosyncrasies of diseases that can affect people. But now that so many are inter-racially marrying and blood lines are mixed, the diseases are not being particular of what blood line you are from anymore.

B. Physical reactions to the drugs taken.

Gary went into the first Chemotherapy session with getting a Hickman Catheter for needles. This was surgically placed under the skin on the upper left side of his chest just under the collar bone. This catheter is a cushion of about 1 inch in diameter and held on a metal frame about 2 inches wide. It is used for a needle with a double port that can be placed in just one time for the entire week's duration of medicines going in, as well as for blood to be drawn out for tests. Tubes from this went into his veins that go out to the body, instead of going into the heart first. He had to have Heparin, a blood thinner, to keep the tube's entrance from clogging. Once this was in, the Chemo treatment seemed to start as uneventful. The shock of finding out about the cancer was still in the forefront of our minds, but this was the first weekend to start the fight against the cancer.

The Outpatient hospital time was about getting the big drugs into Gary's body. When he was at home, he went to bed to rest and get some sleep. At mealtimes, I had to wake him up to eat and specially to drink water. He had to flush the medicine out so it would not stay in his body. He would growl at me to leave him alone, but it had been four hours since he had any water. During the week, he spent an hour at the medical clinic each day with Dr. Yee to get the smaller drugs and normal saline to hydrate his body. She made sure to hydrate him at the hospital after that so he would not have to worry about drinking water. It was a week later that his hair started to fall out from the drugs. Even wiping his moustache with a napkin collected several hairs at a time. When this started, I told him to shave off his moustache so he wouldn't have to deal with it anymore. All of his hair was gone by one month. As he showered, hair went down the drain and had to be unclogged a couple of times.

What was interesting, even though you know that a person doing Chemotherapy will lose their hair, it's still surprising to see that the head is not the only part where it is lost. So are the eyebrows, the moustache (and beard, if a person had one), the underarms, the chest and body hairs, and the legs. Everything. He felt very naked without his normal feeling of hair. A baseball cap became the normal attire with any outfit.

C. Physical appearance and long-term use of the drugs.

Many people going through Chemotherapy will lose weight. As Gary had a hard time eating food, he lost much of his weight in the first two or three months. Since starting with feeling ill, he had dropped 30 or 40 pounds. Dr Yee was actually glad he was slightly overweight to begin with, that he had some weight he could lose. It was jokingly said that this was a fad diet, but not recommended for the general population. The weight continued to drop at the rate of about 10 pounds each month. Having started at about 225 lbs, his low point was at 138 lbs. And he is 6 feet tall. His head seemed to shrink to a small skull without much in the way of skin or fat, or even muscle around the neck. He was stooped because of the surgeries. He walked with a stilted gait because of the shaking caused by the drugs.

What saved me was that this man did not look like my husband. He was a man that I was assigned to take care of and be responsible for. It felt like I knew what Gary would look like at 60 years old, at 80 years old, and maybe at 90 or 100 years old. Thankfully, he does not look like that now. I got my husband mostly back.

The man I played tennis with can no longer run with his shortened lung capacity. He had to train his lungs to expand for deep breaths. He can walk for miles, but not run. The Bleomycin chemicals destroyed not only half of his lungs, but also half of his hearing. He cannot hear the high tones of voices on the telephone and has a difficult time understanding people with heavy accents. The ear ringing, Tinnitus, is a constant companion. The nerve endings in his fingers and toes were also made numb. Dr. Yee recommended he wear gloves in cold weather, or he could get frost bite. And to always wear closed-toed shoes at work, or he would be banging his feet without knowing it. He is not as strong as he used to be in his years of construction, but at least he is his own person again.

The man I married was full of confidence in himself, in his work, and in his mental capacity. I became the one he had to lean on for remembering dates, places, appointments, birthdays, etc. Where he had some patience, he is now more short-tempered, especially with himself. Many times, he can't remember names, but he may remember faces, or maybe can't remember where he had seen someone before. He slowly returned to a more normal level but is still relying on me as a partner to keep things straight. And he still hates doing paperwork, even for his own company.

Please remember that the person you once knew before the illness may not come back as you knew them, either mentally or physically.

You, the caregiver, are assigned for the duration of life, not just the duration of the illness or disease. Try not to think of it as a prison sentence. It won't be if you love him/her. You learn to compromise and change the way you live and think, of what your lives can strive for, and of what your relationship can be for each other. Gary and I take our vacations very seriously ever since he had survived. And it is not "beating" cancer, it is surviving the fight. Illness and disease, whether it be cancer or not, will take its toll on all in the relationship.

D. Food and plastic tableware.

Getting Gary to eat while he was going through Chemotherapy was difficult. He did not want any more after a bite or two—because everything had a flavor of metal. It was the drugs that caused this, but the metal in the forks and spoons seemed like a catalyst and added the metal flavoring to everything he put into his mouth. He found that the plastic tableware did not. At least he could eat without tasting metal.

Food should have been alright to eat if there had not been a physical rejection of it. Everything went in, but much of it came back out. Within fifteen minutes, he would go throw up most of it. It wore him out and he would go to bed to rest, sleep a few hours, and I would wake him up to try again. The only taste that did not seem to change was chocolate. It was a good thing that Ensure Protein drinks came in a chocolate flavor. A can in the hospital was given to him any way he liked. It could be partially frozen for eating like ice cream, again, with a plastic spoon. It could be left alone like a chocolate drink. Or it could be heated like hot chocolate. It was the greatest relief to be able to have something that stayed down. At least it slowed the weight loss a bit.

Trying different things for flavor and tolerance is a long process, but it was worth having the doctor recommend things, like the Ensure Protein drink. Ask your loved one's doctor what they recommend for patients in their condition, as well as how to eat or drink it. It may be faster than trying only on your own.

E. Physical activity.

As Gary became weaker, Dr Yee suggested he walk around the neighborhood for 10 minutes a day to keep up his strength. As he got skinnier and did not look like the Gary everyone knew, the neighbors thought I was walking with my father or grandfather. We could not do this on the days he was in the hospital. He tried as many times as was possible. My problem was that he was shuffling in his walk. After the surgery and several chemotherapy sessions, he would step up on the sidewalk or stair with one foot and drag his other foot, forgetting he was stepping up and, thereby, tripping.

Gary's perception of distance was off. It scared me that he might trip and fall when I was not near to catch his arm. The medical clinic I worked at was adding an extension of another two-story building alongside the old building. The Oncology appointment was on the second floor. A closet next to the elevator of the old building would be used for another elevator to go completely from the basement to the second floor of the new building. A hole was being dug on each floor. We stepped out of the old elevator, and I headed to the reception desk to check in. I turned and saw Gary reaching out with his arm to lean on an opposite wall so he could look down into the hole of the floor. The construction caution tape was lying on the floor, and he had stepped over it. I could foresee him falling head-first down three floors. With my heart in my throat with fear, I hurried to him and pulled his arm, dragging him across pneumatic hoses on the floor.

"Would you please not go into the construction area!" I whispered harshly at him.

"Let go of my arm!" he replied as he tripped on the hoses, "I just wanted to see it!" He and his family had construction in their careers. It was his natural curiosity that I believed would kill him!

"You're not supposed to do that here!" He was mad at me for some time.

My father was taking care of my mother during her dementia. As she became incapable of dressing, going to the bathroom, and doing ordinary things, like eating and bathing herself, Dad took over. His problem was that she was walking all the time, inside and outside. He would take her to the shopping malls and park way in the back. He walked her around for a couple of hours for her to get tired enough to go home and have a nap. Most times, she didn't even nap after walking, it was just that he had to go to the bathroom and took her home for the both of them to go.

A friend watched over his wife as she was going through Chemotherapy, who also had lots of energy. She had a stationary bike to pedal away hours when she felt jittery and twitchy from the chemicals. It was unfortunate that the type of cancer she had was something different and rare. She died a couple years later, even after the experimental drugs from City of Hope.

Another friend had a husband that was not supposed to strain his facial muscles with lifting heavy objects. He had plastic surgery on his face after his cancer had eaten away part of his jaw's facial muscle coverage. He loved working on his racing cars and lifted body parts or engine parts. This would tear up his face with the plastic surgery again before it had healed for a few years. After his Chemotherapy, she had to force him to have a friend or family member help do these things for him while he watched impatiently. And because he could not go to work, he was under her feet when she came home from her work, while she was cooking dinner, and when she was trying to clean house and do laundry. He was too impatient to help with these chores, only getting half done at any one time. He finally was let back to work, but they had to monitor how much he lifted.

As a caregiver, you will have to watch for the changes that happen to your loved one.

Watch that their physical actions are not impaired in their normal movements. If they still recognize that they need to do things, it might have to be told, not asked, to get dressed, bathe, and eat. You, of course, will be told to go to hell, but it still needs to be said.

Chapter 2 – The Mental Aspect
A. At the doctors, and the wall comes down.

The first Oncology appointment with Dr. Yee was quite different from any ordinary doctor appointment I had ever been to. I was used to being asked how I am feeling. What have I done to take care of myself with a cold? What did I eat that is making me feel bad? Certainly not an appointment of a doctor asking Gary if he had been having strange and vivid dreams. If he had been waking up sweating for no reason. Had he been able to keep any food down? Was he short with his temper to all who were around him?

Before doing the gastroscopy, the x-ray of Gary's abdomen showed that he had mal-rotated intestines. Perhaps 1 person in 100,000 have this fairly rare physical difference. His appendix was behind his navel. His intestines move down, instead of to the left, then to the right and around. The slices of MRI pictures Dr. Yee showed us had a tumor that looked to be the size of a large turnip where there should have been an empty cavity around the organs. As I described before, the "root" of this tumor went around Gary's kidneys and intestines, and the "stem" of it went up and was headed for his heart and lungs. The bulk of this tumor was leaning on the large intestine where the scopes had been stopped and closed the intestine to where it was blocking any passage of digested food. The reason the exploratory surgery was stopped was so not even a capillary would be nicked and allow cancer cells to enter Gary's bloodstream.

Sitting there listening to Dr. Yee, this is where I almost physically saw a block wall, like a heavy, solid garage door, go down in front of Gary's face. He would not comprehend anything else that the doctor was saying. He was through listening to any more about this tumor, or cancer, or anything else. I had to listen to the doctor and of her plan to combat this thing.

Gary was in Stage 3, where Stage 4 is terminal. He had a 10% chance of surviving at that point. She laid out the chemicals that would be needed to fight the cancer cells, and the surgery needed to get rid of the tumor once the tendrils had been driven back down, giving the statistic that this combination would be a possible success. It was his best chance to survive the cancer and the Chemotherapy. She did say "survive the cancer," not "beat the cancer." In the old days, they called cancer by the name of Consumption. It consumed the body.

Should the doctor do the treatment, or not? When some people have been told a "dooms day" threat like this, there are many who would deny that it could be that bad. They are strong and would not be struck down by a small cancer cell. Some patients do not want treatment because they think it will all work out and go away. Or the opposite effect might happen, where the patient is convinced that he/she will die whether with or without any help by Chemotherapy or surgery. It has been chosen by God to let the cancer take its course and die when it is time. Others seem to try everything.

There are no two patients alike. But if the patient won't listen, it is up to the caregiver to handle what needs to be decided.

Each individual is unique. The caregiver will need to figure out the best course of action and go with it. Knowing the statistics of the most common outcome will help make that decision.

B. The world of pain is only their arm's length.

Uncle Rich was going through prostate cancer when Aunt Sally asked me why he was acting so strange. He had his Chemotherapy and all his medicines, as well as morphine. Whenever he wanted, at the push of a little button, he could get a dose because it was hooked to his IV (intravenous) Drip.

"I know he loves me," Aunt Sally complained, "but he is

constantly yelling at me about anything and everything. What did I do?"

I explained that she had not done anything wrong. She was taking care of him as was her duty as a wife. She helped him from the beginning of the day until the end of the day. But she happened to be within range of his world of pain. When a person is in constant pain, it narrows the person's focus to just their personal space. **They are aware of the world by only the length of their arms around them.**

Whoever is caring for the ill person will naturally come within this range and get the brunt of the anger and frustration of not getting rid of it.

With Gary in constant pain, I was called all kinds of names, even though he tried not to yell at me. He apologized when he realized he had shouted at me in annoyance of telling him to drink more water, or to lift his feet better when walking, or trying to button shirts by himself and I was trying to help. As the Chemo would let up for a few days, he would be frustrated that it was not over with yet. By the next weekend, his blood platelets would be too low and start the 100F degree fever. Off to the hospital again for another blood transfusion of a couple pints. Gary was asked if he would like Regular or Ethyl. Ethyl, please.

C. Change of personality.

It is devastating to learn that your loved one is going through an illness that could possibly be fatal. What also is a shock is the possible change in character and mental attitude of your loved one. Most patients do a 180-degree turnaround of mentality and personality change.

What was once an outspoken, outgoing person, my husband was now a recluse refusing to go anywhere or do anything outside of doctor visits and hospital stays. He did not want people to see him as he was or talk to anyone that might find out he was ill. He growled at me anytime I tried to get him to do something or go anywhere.

It was like he wanted to crawl into a corner and die. He would go to sleep and try not to wake up, so he would not have to deal with the world. He said it was because he was worn out with not sleeping the whole night through and the sleep was the only brief relief he could get.

My mother was a physical therapist with healing in her hands. Doctors would send her people who had been in car accidents. One man was half paralyzed and was walking with a walker within six months, where the doctors had warned him that he may never walk again. When my mother began her slow journey in dementia, she began hallucinating that the gofers in the back yard were Lilliputians from Gulliver's Travels, and that the dog was giving them rides on his back. My father said that as long as she did not involve him, he was fine with her actions. She changed to an angry woman within three years. It was when she insisted that he help a broken-down car in front of their house, when there was nothing there, he called for a Social Services interview to determine if she would need any medication. It happened that the nurse to do the interview arrived at the same time that my mother was swinging a broom at my father. She was yelling that he was not willing to help anyone with car trouble anymore. The nurse was nodding her head. Yes, my mother needed medication.

A friend has a roommate sharing a large apartment. He and his wife were good friends, and his wife was close to my friend's daughter. The wife suddenly became confrontational and hostile, coming nose-to-nose to my friend with threats that she could "get her" if she wanted. It was like a window of a house within her mind where a different angry room was visible. She had to call her roommate to calm his wife down with loving talk. When the window of this other angry personality closed, she would retreat back into the house in her mind. That was the signal to them that something else was going on besides the headaches she was experiencing. She was diagnosed with a brain tumor. Her appetite decreased so badly that when the window opened up that she was hungry, a plate of food was made. But by the time it was made and set before her, a bite or two was all that was eaten as she twirled it around with her spoon or fork. The window of hunger had closed. Then she complained that she was not hungry, and why had they made so much food? The roommate had to help his wife with her clothes, going to the bathroom, and almost force feed her. He had to calmly talk her down whenever she was angry with the world when that window of anger from within her mind was showing through. It was unfortunate that she died within six months.

D. Why me?

A difficult part of the caring process is trying to answer the questions that the ill person keeps asking. Why me? What did I do to deserve this? Haven't I been good enough that I don't need to suffer this way?

For Gary, my answer to him was that had he not had mal-rotated intestines, we would not have found out about the tumor for another month or two before going to see a doctor. He was lucky to have this added time advantage to fight this cancer. Of course, he did not deserve to suffer, and that is why Dr. Yee had several things that helped with the Chemo. She gave him pain pills and shots, nausea medicines, tranquillizing pills, sleeping pills, and anything else she could think of. This is one thing Dr. Yee believed that the patient need not suffer from aches and pains while doing Chemotherapy. There were other things Gary had to think about, like trying to do work at the shop with his mother's help.

The caregiver has to find a unique way to answer the questions.

Try to find what was good about his/her illness that would have killed another person in the family more quickly. Or that the Chemo is working as fast as it can, under the circumstances. Or that the time needed for treatments are now halfway through. Something that is relevant to you and your loved one.

E. I can still drive the car!

One of the mental and physical mixtures is when the loved one insists that they can still do the things they normally do, even though the Chemotherapy has impaired their judgment.

Gary insisted on driving to one of his appointments with Dr Yee. It was in January about six weeks into his treatments. As it was for a 10 a.m. appointment, I thought it was safe enough to let him. We first went to a café for breakfast. He almost ran over the tire stop for parking. It was a surprise to both of us that he hit the stop forcibly enough to bounce the car up a bit. As we ate, he asked how he was doing. Ok, I guess. He drove the rest of the way to the clinic, just a little bit early, and he asked me again how I thought he had done.

"Well," I started, "you did fine with your steering, speed, and braking. As you could see from your parking at the café, your depth perception is slightly off."

"What do you mean?"

"Ok. Well, at the stop light, the one where you actually had to stop, you were beyond the crosswalk and into the intersection. Luckily, no traffic was coming from the other way, and you could go again without any incident. Had there been a car, they would have had to swerve around the nose of our car to get around us. Maybe it would be better if I drive to the doctors and hospital for a while. Just until you get better again and can drive like you normally do." The protests came.

Gary did not want to give up driving, but for safety's sake, I pleaded to let me drive until he was done with the Chemotherapy. Hopefully, you, the caregiver, will not have to argue about whether their driving ability is still safe. Try to say that you are going for their moral support and use this excuse to do the driving.

F. Don't give me that stuff! I don't want it! I want to go home!

Anyone who has had an injured muscle can tell you that it is tiring to keep doing therapy on those muscles to get them right. It took a year for my dislocated shoulder to go from a one-inch movement in any direction to full motion. But I was persistent with doing the exercises to do a full circle of the arm.

It is the same with taking medicines over and over and over again. Chemotherapy for Gary took a long time to get through. After the first weekend of major drugs pumped into Gary's body, four days of minor drugs pumped in at the doctor's office, and a week or so for the drugs to take effect, his blood platelets went to less than 100 white cell count and less than 1000 red cell count in a unit of blood. Normal is 350 to 500 white cells and 5000 to 7000 red cells. When the fever spiked to over 100F degrees, he returned to the hospital to get a refill.

Another two or three days in the hospital. We figured that he went through 13 complete oil changes (of blood), and his mileage was not very good. He couldn't go three weeks without more.

Each month, Gary had blood drawn to send to a Connecticut laboratory for his tumor marker. Yes, the tumor marker is also a pregnancy test, but with more detail. Can you imagine that a woman pregnant with a child, that it is also considered a tumor? The difference is that the baby has a heartbeat. The cancer tumor does not. The marker seemed to tell us the cancer cells were cut in half each time, but it got slower as the tumor got smaller.

Each time we made another Chemotherapy trip to the hospital, Gary would try to talk Dr. Yee into letting him go home earlier than was scheduled. Dr. Yee had an interesting answer: "We'll see." She would have to see what the blood tests were doing with his blood refills and check to see that no infections were creeping up into his body. If more or different drugs were needed, she could get it into him before he left. She never promised anything, but gave him the discerning eye and told him, "We'll see."

It was me that he shouted at that he did not want any more of that stuff. He had enough already, why can't he go home? So my answer became: "We'll see what Dr. Yee says." He scoffed at me that I was no help, and I was taking her side, not his. I said, "Yeah, we'll see."

If needed, a caregiver can also use this answer to ward off arguments from the loved one. "We'll see if the doctor can eliminate (this or that) drug this time." "We'll see if you can go to (here or there)." "We'll see if you can do that, or not." It's not a promise and it's not an argument. It's an open suggestion that you and they will try something to see if it will work, or not. You'll see.

G. Talk about plans for the future.

Much of anyone's plans for the future will change dramatically when a loved one becomes acutely ill or die. In my mind, I watched my plans for a European vacation go out the window. I was enrolled to take a French class at Mt. San Antonio College. I barely got out of it before classes started. I don't know if I will get to go now. When Gary was depressed about how his body was doing, he wanted to just roll over and die. I had to start talking about the travels we still wanted to do, places we wanted to go. I still wanted him to be with me to do all that. I wanted our kids to see some of the places, too. We have, thankfully, done some of our travels and have taken the kids traveling. There are still places we want to see. We may still get to go to Europe, although now it will be in the retirement years.

My father watched as his dream of becoming a self-employed, part-time welder after he retired from his 8 to 5 job go out the window. He had to take care of my mother as she began her slow, dark journey of dementia.

He spent three years of caring for Mom at home, five years of seeing her every day at the nursing center, and two years of sitting by her side or wheeling her about in a wheelchair. She passed away at 63. Dad, then 70, moved into a 55+ living apartment. He had people he could talk to about the old wars and the old days. When he became ill, he moved in with my brother. He stayed there for several years, then went into an assisted living complex for a few years. He passed away at 82.

A co-worker saw his life go out the window when his wife committed suicide in a state of low depression. He had three small children to care for. He could not even think about a far-off future, so I suggested a few things for the immediate future. He could trade his computer skills for people who had offered to help. I also let him know to limit the time that they would be doing something for him, say for the next two weeks, could they take his oldest child to school until he could get more permanent arrangements.

Always give an ending date so that people, who offered to do anything at all for you, will have the feeling of accomplishment, rather than feeling like they are stuck for life at a task.

This would help give this father time to think about what needed to be done first, like the funeral, babysitting, and having grandparents help, if they could. He needed to take time each day to sit and cry with his kids where they would not feel left out. He had to assure them that Mommy was not mad at them. He can look further to the future after they had all settled down. And he needed to keep his job to continue earning money for their livelihood.

You, the caregiver, will need to look at what changes will need to take place, where former activities, dreams, and accomplishments were set aside. Think of what can still be done or what still can be accomplished after the illness or death.

Without future goals, the loved one will not have a light at the end of the tunnel to look forward to.

It was a statistic that gave me hope for Gary to live: Those that had to fight for their life did better when a loved one and/or family were pulling for them. They still had something to live for. Give your loved one something to strive for to get moving in the healthy direction if you can.

H. Talk to the children.

My boys were 6 and 9 years old while Gary was battling the cancer. The youngest was in kindergarten, the oldest in third grade. I visited the kindergarten class and let the teacher know that I might have to hurry and take my son out of the class if I had to take Gary to the hospital before a school day was done. She said she would never have known had I not told her what was going on.

My oldest was troubled with his classmates constantly asking how his dad was doing. When did they give him medicine? Was he getting any better? Is he out of the hospital? He was crying when I was tucking him into bed on a weekend where I actually saw my kids in the evening. I asked if he wanted to talk about it and he told me what was going on at school. He did not mind telling the others what news he had, but it was tiring to keep repeating himself. The other kids were his friends, so I suggested he tell one person, then tell the others to ask that person instead of repeating himself. Just tell the rest that you didn't want to talk about it anymore, but they could go ask so-and-so if they wanted.

My son also told me that he was scared he would really lose his father. So was I and I let him know that. He wanted to take a shotgun and just shoot the cancer out of Dad's body. I explained that was exactly what the Chemotherapy medicines were doing to his dad. Each time Dad did the Chemo, it was a battle to see who would not be destroyed the most. The good blood cells, or the bad cancer cells. We just hoped that the good blood cells would win out. My son asked how long it would take to get rid of the cancer cells. With a sigh, I told him we had to keep doing this until there were no more cancer cells left to fight. We did not really know how long that would take. We cried together a bit more until he went to sleep.

You, the caregiver, not only have to take care of the loved one with the illness or disability, but also the rest of the family. Some children will not be able to understand what is going on. My youngest knew his dad was ill, but not that it could be fatal. My oldest caught on very quickly that it was a very serious fight with cancer. Don't try to hide any information from the child that does understand why a parent is constantly going to the hospital. If they ask questions, just answer them as honestly as you can at their level.

Kids are a lot smarter than you think.

It was easy to explain that we had to be very careful with cleaning everything and helping Dad get around. Both of my boys cooperated as much as they could without a fuss or argument.

Chapter 3 – The Social Aspect
A. Don't tell anyone.

I know that I don't feel like visiting with friends and family while I am sick. I don't look well, and usually there is the reason that I don't want to spread the germs to anyone else to become sick. Gary had this same feeling about himself, that he did not look his best, and he didn't have the energy to visit anyone for more than 10 minutes. Plus, he did not want anyone to know he was so sick to maybe dying and get their pity that he was ill. It was not feeling sorry for himself. It was a prevention of not wanting to see people's faces when they were saying they were so sorry for him to have to fight this.

There were family members and cousins around Gary that knew what he had to do with surgeries or about being stuck in bed. Others left him alone with hardly a call to see if he was doing better or not. Most of his friends had no idea about this fight with cancer, because Gary insisted that we don't tell anyone. He wanted to wait until he was better before talking about it. Not even his oldest friends that he still talked to would know about his fight with cancer until after it was over. Either he would be dead, or he had survived.

Although Gary insisted that we not tell anyone, several people did find out about his cancer. They stayed away to not be involved. He lost a couple of these fair-weather friends, but he could not be rid of his own brother. Rick did not like hospitals and doctors, and he thought Gary's doctor was not doing a very good job. He needed a second opinion, so why was Gary not searching for another doctor?

After Rick had left, Gary was crying when I came in before going to work. I became angry. Gary not only had a second opinion, but also a third, a fourth, and a fifth opinion. Gary had an Oncologist that was a professor teaching at USC Medical Center. Even her husband is a professor at USC. Gary had a highly rated Urologist, two excellent surgeons, and a General

Practitioner that gladly asked for others' opinions. If you as a caregiver have any feelings like the doctor is not doing all he/she can for your loved one, it is highly recommended even by other doctors that you should check out their credentials as a doctor. I was lucky to be associated with so many good ones.

Don't let anyone tell you that you are not doing all you can for your loved one. It is more than that complaining person would probably be willing to do themselves.

As I stated before, each person is different, and each case is different. It will keep peace if you do as your loved one wishes. In my opinion, telling just a few people would be fine. I don't believe telling the whole world that your loved one is fighting the big fight will help. With social media being used as a big thing, it is hard not to use it. I still suggest keeping it private. Unless, of course, you want to have the whole world knowing about it. This is a decision between you and your loved one.

B. Dressing for an occasion.

Clothes can be a challenge to all involved in getting dressed. As the loved one becomes thinner, the clothes are not usually replaced, simply because there really is no time to do shopping for clothes when all are hoping for recovering from the illness. It's just that the weight loss can be very dramatic, and the ill person wants to think they will survive and will fit right back into their clothes.

As the progression of Chemotherapy took its toll on Gary's body, I watched as his clothes began to hang loosely on him. His belt would show more holes as he went down another notch to tighten the grip of his pants. He looked like a little kid in his daddy's big clothes. Dr. Yee suggested he get some new clothes that fit him. He refused because he would be getting better and fit back into them. Why should he buy another wardrobe for just a few months? He finally relented and got a pair of pants with an elastic waistband. It was still big as he got his normal size pants, but it was able to look like it would stay up. The caregiver will be dressing some or all of the clothes on a loved one as the illness drags on. We found that elastic-waisted pants worked well for ease of dressing up or down. Velcro strapped shoes were much quicker to handle with moving feet. And flatter walking shoes at that. Hats or a baseball cap made the baldness of the head seem less striking to see. It might not be a problem nowadays, where so many people like having a shaved head. Hats also keep them warm and dry in the wind or rain. If it is extremely cold, gloves on the hands and slip-on boots help keep fingers and toes from freezing.

My Mom did not really know how to explain that her fingers were cold, but we could feel how cold she was getting. Dad learned that he should dress as he wanted her to be dressed. Mom had the exact number of layers of clothing as he did. If he got hot, he would take off a coat or sweater and, in turn, take off a coat or sweater from Mom.

Take a hint: Dress the same layers of clothes on your loved one as you would have on.

Take off your sweater and his/her sweater at the same time so you know what temperature you are dealing with, whether inside or outside. Shoes, not sandals, should be closed-toed and comfortable for all day walking and for protecting feet from stubbing toes and tripping. And for women, no high heels, please. They should be flat enough to not stumble.

C. Reverse Isolation, wearing a mask.

One of the hardest experiences I had was when Gary caught pneumonia and stayed in the hospital for a full two weeks. He was at his lowest weight, his immune system was way down, and he just didn't seem to have enough blood in his body to fight anything off. Here we thought the cancer would be the one to kill him when pneumonia was the real threat.

My time schedules were completely rearranged with twice

daily trips to the hospital, keeping the kids going in and out of school, and staying at my job to keep the insurance paying for most of this. With many lines attached to Gary, he was not able to take a shower. An IV in the port, oxygen in his nose, and sometimes a urine catheter was a constant hospital protocol.

Sponge baths were the only way to be clean, which I gave him, so a strange nurse would not be doing it. That was one of the things that Gary did not like. He only saw a nurse for about three days, another would show up for three or four days, and yet another would show up for three days. Looking as bad as he felt he looked, he did not want so many people being familiar with his body. It was just a "pet peeve," so I did it.

Isolation is when a patient stays away from all people and everything in a room that is sterile. **Reverse Isolation** is when anyone coming into Gary's sterilized room must be gowned up. Because of all the tubes in his way, Gary could not wear a mask. And with his immune system so low, it meant that any and all doctors, nurses, and visitors were required to put on a full gown, head covering, mask, gloves, and booties over the shoes. No germ was supposed to be able to get near him.

At this point, it was not so much that the cancer was a threat as any germ that could invade his body and run rampant, pneumonia being a very severe one. It was a week of antibiotics and oxygen before this critical episode allowed us to again visit without looking like operating room interns.

The second week of this hospital stay was so that his blood could be refilled, as well as to see that the pneumonia was gone. They also watched to see that he could breathe on his own again.

Near the end of the week, Gary's father and his cousins came to visit him, all standing next to his bed, talking with him, joking around, trying to keep Gary's attitude up with a smile. Near the foot end of the bed where I stood, the blanket looked like it was wrinkled up. I thought to straighten it out just for something to do. As I was about to reach down to pull the blanket straight, the wrinkle moved. It was Gary's leg! He had lost so much weight that the bones seemed to be all that was left of him! I started to shake and hyperventilate from the shock. I had to get out of the room to breathe. As I stood in the hall leaning against the wall, my father-in-law came out and asked if I was all right. All I could do was shake my head and try not to break down. I took slow deep breathes to calm down.

Fighting the cancer is a struggle, but germs and bacteria have a way of being transmitted by air as well as by touch and can invade a weakened body very easily. It is often started with someone in the family having a common cold. As I said, the pneumonia was the real threat to the health of the patient. Even at home, I was cleaning everything with bleach and antibacterial soaps so Gary would not get sick.

Remember to wash doors and doorknobs; walls where people's hands touch; handrails where people grab going up or down stairways; the kitchen counters and faucets; the bathroom sink, toilet, and tub; and anything else that is touched by the family and your loved one.

Even with being as careful as I was, Gary still got a cold and it quickly worked into pneumonia.

D. Wearing a mask at home with visitors.

It was difficult for Gary to walk, or stand, or sit in an uncomfortable chair while visiting with anyone, so we did not make any effort to go out. With Christmas, several friends and family were visiting our house. What to do about other people's germs? Gary wore a mask for protection. He sat in his comfortable reclining chair in the living room, which was set away from the draft of the front door and sliding glass door to the outside. A blanket was on the arm against the cold, and everyone could sit on the sofa or at the dining room table for conversation. No one was allowed to touch Gary unless they had used a hand sanitizer. Gary felt very self-conscience about this, but it was the only way to keep him safe. It is acceptable now to replace the handshake with the fist bump (after being sanitized).

Using a mask around an ill person is a safeguard against many germs. Whether visiting at home or at the hospital, the one ill person or the many visitors should be wearing one. And anyone with a cold or cough should be considerate enough to wear one all the time around people in general.

Cleaning and disinfecting doorknobs are an easy way to cut down on germs being spread to others. Many people love to use bleach. I would love to use bleach more often, but my brand is Lysol Disinfectant that also kills 99% of germs and Comet (with bleach!) for scrubbing.

Besides using masks, you will also have to try different things to see how your loved one will handle smells.

The smell of bleach throws Gary into a flashback to all the hospital stays he experienced. I try to minimize that.

Chapter 4 – Psychological/Spiritual Aspect
A. Getting nice things your loved one always wanted to give you.

When Gary proposed marriage to me on the Lover's Lot, an empty lot that overlooked the city, he wanted to give me the world. He couldn't give me the full moon looking down on us because he couldn't reach it, but he could maybe put a toll gate on the freeway below if I wanted. Of course, I said yes.

We had been going out for two and a half years, steady for one of them. There was no other man that I could compare to for what Gary meant to me, because he rated very well for my list of qualities I wanted in a man. He was my equal in education. He had an almost photographic memory and intellect. He had common sense and even thought philosophically as I did. He did the same things that I was doing even before we met, both of us being active in high school and college tennis, and karate. And we listened to the same music; therefore, the double record albums in our collection. He was my best friend. We meshed together very naturally. It was logical and natural that we get married.

As the cancer ate away at Gary's body, the goals that he had in his mind were being eaten away by the possible lack of time that he now had on this earth. With two kids, there is not very much spare, expendable cash flow allowed in the daily living of house and home. He still wanted to give me beautiful things and take me to beautiful places. We bought timeshares, as it was similar in cost to staying at a hotel. Our boys were raised with a swimming pool at these places and got to alternately see Disneyland, Sea World, San Diego Zoo, and San Diego Wild Animal Park each year. It was not enough. Gary still wanted our trip to Europe, which his father and brother did. He wanted to show me the place of his ancestors in England and Ireland. He wanted to take me to Holland to see my place of birth once more. This was not going to happen if he died.

The replacement of all these dreams began to show up in expensive jewelry, perfumes, fancy clothes, and fabulous dining out. Thank you, God, for the credit cards you allowed me to handle. I tried to curb fancy clothes and dining out to once a month, one special outfit or outing. And it was not just Gary and I that went out. It was for the whole family, and it's double the expense. At Christmas, gold bracelets and expensive perfumes came in.

How could we afford all this? My work, Gary's work, and his Disability Insurance managed to handle it all. My mother-in-law asked how I could keep all this if Gary died. I told her I would have returned the gold bracelets because I would not be able to handle the payments anymore. I would have to negotiate with the credit card companies for a lower payment plan with the cards being closed for no further purchases. And I would have to arrange to sell Gary's business and shop equipment to get rid of the expense as no more income would be coming from it. It was not a pretty picture and was extra stress to me.

It took years of steady income and steady paying of bills for our life to continue even past the cancer fight. I had to let Gary know that he was with me on this budget and could not go to any extravagance anymore. He understood it and went back to work at his shop. We were in this together and we had to work together to keep what we had.

If this happens to you, try to make sure that your budget can handle any extra expenses brought on by your loved one. If it can't, then try to tell him/her that it is not possible to keep whatever he/she is trying to give you. We also had a car payment, so if your loved one tries to give you a car that you can't keep, try to explain that the money is just not there for the payments, if it isn't already a payment that has to be made on your current car. It might be one of the harder things to argue about. It may bring on tears of frustration that your loved one cannot "just give you something nice," but you absolutely cannot let it break your bank account. You still need a place to live, sleep, and eat.

B. Being too generous.

It was probably a good thing that I was with Gary whenever he went out of the house. Every time we went to a place other than the doctor's office or the hospital, there was some good cause for someone on the street, or in the store, or charity that was going on, and Gary wanted to donate money. At least I could restrict it to the money he had in his wallet. No credit cards were allowed. No late-night TV and donating to third world countries no matter how cute and sad Sally's face was. We had our own struggles first. Then, later, after all this was over, we could think about donating to others.

If you can, keep your loved one from donating your lives away. It is very hard to restrict the credit card use, but show him/her the bills that come in.

You have a budget you must keep and these need to be looked at by both of you.

Teamwork on the finances will help if you can get him/her to see it.

C. God doesn't love me anymore.

I have always felt that I am a beacon, or a vessel, that Jesus' light from above shines through me and onto the world. Gary and I are Christians, but we are not religious. We like to show by example how the world should be treated. We offer many organizations our services or goods. Donations are made wherever needed and can do best for those that need it. Gary felt like he had been a good Christian, but he still got this cancer. Why did he have to get it? Was he not to be with his family? "God doesn't love me anymore."

This was at Gary's lowest level of illness, both physically and mentally. He did not want to do the extra surgery to remove the tumor that had been shrunk down. It was my argument that God had helped in shrinking the tumor so that it could be removed. That was why this surgery was needed. Being reminded that the surgery would be like having a baby by C-section, he did not want to do this, at all. Yes, it was like having a baby, but this thing had to be removed so that any hiding live cancer cells could not flare up again. I talked until my face was blue to get him to do this. And yes, it was like having a C-section baby, but this baby was for the trash. No heart was beating in it, and no amount of Chemotherapy could kill all the cells that needed to be killed.

After the surgery, tests were done to see if there was anything going on inside the tumor. And yes, there were live cells in the tumor that would have made a come-back. A couple of cleanup Chemo sessions would do the trick of getting the last of the cancer cells in his body. My argument was that this surgery was needed. God made the opportunity to get rid of the tumor, and we had taken that step as intended. Gary is still with his family. I think God still loves him.

You and your loved one may get into arguments about how to go about the treatments needed to help cure the illness, or to help your environment to accommodate the changes needed. Use the same argument that no other person in your family or friends would have been able to go through what he/she had just been through.

Go with what your faith suggests doing. Both of you should agree from the beginning that your God will guide you.

As a caregiver, it was my part to argue for the surgery. It may also be your part. It depends on what you and your loved one believe should happen. So, help it to happen the way it should. And do lots of praying.

Chapter 5 – Advocate & Document Keeper

A. Advocate for the patient

Every ill person needs a voice, an advocate to make sure that needs are met, that comfort is given, and that the accommodations are comfortable. An advocate fights for the loved one to get the treatments needed and does all the background work that the ill person cannot do. And the advocate is usually the caregiver.

You, the caregiver, need to be the advocate for your loved one.

I argued with the hospital for charges not needed. I argued with insurance companies that would not cover certain unapproved items. I argued with doctors and nurses to get what was needed by Gary, the patient. And I argued with Gary to do the things and actions needed to fight this cancer. Medical bills, as complicated as that, is why an advocate is needed.

When my mother-in-law had been in the Nursing facility with a breathing machine, she could not speak until later when they put the oxygen tube in her throat. To get a nurse's attention, she sometimes threw a hairbrush into the hall, or a small stuffed toy that our son had given her. The nurse would come in, curious and a bit irritated that Mom was throwing things at them. Only then did they find that the Nurse Call button on the long cord was on her pillow above her head where she could not reach it.

We sometimes came in to see her and found it again out of her reach. We had to tell the nurses to check in on her after her sponge bath to see that she could get to the Nurse Call button. At the time, Mom had no way to tell the nurses what she wanted. Things as simple as that, is why an advocate is needed.

B. Finding out about the illness and what you can do.

Once the doctors explained what was happening to Gary's body, it was up to me to find out what they were talking about. Looking up information then was different in that

I had to go to the library to look up books and read pamphlets that the doctors could give us. Now, anyone can Google search any ailment, ache, and pain. There is an explanation on the internet out there that will help with what you need to know. I had to rely on the doctors to tell me what was expected of both the chemicals and the body reactions that might happen. It surprised me when people asked how Gary was doing and I could explain from a medical point of view of what was happening. I had gained knowledge that an ordinary person would not usually learn about.

By putting my mind in this learning mode, it helped to know what to expect from not only the cancer, but also what chemicals were needed to combat it. With Gary, chemicals were used in a shotgun effect, where good cells as well as bad cells were destroyed. The internal fight was to see what survived, the good or the bad. When my mother-in-law had lung cancer, a pinpoint two-laser attack was set at 90-degree angles to destroy the cancer cell. So now, only the bad cells could be blasted instead of entire sections of good and bad cells being hit.

You may now be allowed to feel like a nurse.

The caregiver needs to know about the illness and what chemicals will be used, and how it will affect the loved one. Find out what the after-effects the chemicals do to the body, and what will remain intact if all goes well. This also strengthens your mind, from a medical point of view, to deal with the illness. It helps move some of the personal effect to the side where you can discuss the illness and explain to other family members what is going on.

C. Insurance & Financial fighting.

The bills started coming at me from the second week and never seemed to stop. I had to set up a box with folders to keep everything straight. One section was for the doctor visits, the others for hospital visits. As each bill came in, the notations on it said the clinic had sent in the bills to the insurance company. I was to wait until the insurance had paid or told us that it was denied. As I had said earlier, there was a point where I had 24 visits to the hospital in one year. Each bill was for either Chemotherapy treatment or blood refills. Oh, and the long pneumonia hospital stay.

Insurance paid for their 80% of the approved invoice. After the insurance paid their portion, the balance is due by the patient. There always seemed to be something that they did not approve. I had to call and argue with them for things the doctor had ordered but was not on their list of approved coverage. As I wrote a check out for several bills at once, I had to write each account number and how much to put towards it. Each check I wrote was about $100.00 to $150.00 paying for ten to fifteen bills. I was paying $10.00 to each bill. It is unbelievable that it took five years to pay off all the hospital bills. It was like doing a car payment.

At six months, I started to get calls from the hospital threatening to turn over Gary's bills to a collection agency. I asked them to look at the check # and how much the check was for. And look up Gary's name instead of an account number. I was paying what I could at the $10.00 per account so that I could keep each account active. "Oh!" was the reaction I got for months as the calls came.

Sometimes, the insurance bill will show charges that may be wrong or doubled. Call the insurance company and ask if this bill is accurate. Don't be afraid to ask why one thing or another on the list is not being covered. I became angry when I saw they charged $3.95 for an aspirin. Was Gary buying a whole bottle? Besides, wasn't Gary supposed to have pain shots? Not aspirins! The next time, I brought a bottle of aspirins from home, just in case. It was taken off the bill.

You, the caregiver, will have to keep all the accounts in their file slot so you can remember to pay only once per month on each account. By paying only $10.00 per account, the hospital wants to keep your money coming in. I told them there is no way I can pay an account off because of the other accounts, and I could not afford any more than what is sent in. You may be in the same situation, where you can only send in as much as you can afford.

D. Keeping records.

By law, all personal financial records must be kept for at least three years and business records are kept for seven years. I have a shredding day once each year to get rid of the oldest year back. Keep all records needed in a place where you can easily get to them. By having them in a file drawer, it can easily and quickly be put into a car if a fire disaster forces you to evacuate your home.

When medical records are needed for income tax time, remember that it will not be able to be done online on a simple E-form.

This is more complicated and will need to be calculated as to how much of your medical payments can be taken off your income tax. As this is on forms that are not handled online, you will have to send in the paper forms. If you cannot figure out how to do all this, a reputable income tax company can help. Yes, you will have to pay for their services, but it may be worth it to be accurate. Insurance papers are needed to keep a record of how much they have covered for the hospital visit, doctor visit, labs, x-rays, and pharmaceutical charges. These should also be kept in a file drawer for safe keeping for three years.

Chapter 6 – Self Aspect of the Caregiver
A. Keeping your own body healthy.

When I found myself getting exhausted, I took a multi-vitamin with iron to give me a boost. I don't normally need extra iron, usually taking vitamins without it, and it's tough for me to take more than one a week as it constipates me. If you find yourself getting exhausted, ask your own doctor if you should take something extra to keep going. If you are on any medications, also ask your doctor if it would be safe or not for you to take iron with your multi-vitamins. I also tried to be at full capacity with my Vitamin C so I would not get sick.

In the morning, I would start the day with a set of vitamins so I could keep up with everything during the day. There is an invisible rule that mothers are not allowed to get sick. I did not know how I would survive financially if I did not go to work to keep the insurance paying for all the bills. I couldn't afford to get sick. I worked from 5 p.m. to 11 p.m. at a medical clinic. After getting the kids home and starting dinner, I got in my shower and got ready for work. After brushing my teeth, I took another set of vitamins with a big glass of water. As I got home late, everyone was in bed sleeping, but I was still wound up. With headphones on I did my exercises in the living room. I did this for a year and a half. The exercising was a stress reliever for me, and I would get tired enough to go to bed. Maybe this would be a stress reliever for you.

With all the stress of going on and on, I found myself losing a lot of hair in my hairbrush. It concerned me that I might be empathizing with Gary at his hair loss! My hairdresser told me, no, it was just the stress for my part. But she asked me if I massaged my head at all. I asked why. She explained that if my skin is taut from my being tense, it can remain that way if not massaged. I found that I had to massage my forehead as well for keeping away the headaches. My hairdresser was happy to see new hairs growing where it had started to get thin. I started to thin out again when I had lost my job years later and was stressed out. I remembered her advice and again had to massage my head to get the skin to move. I don't lose very much hair now.

As you shower and wash your hair, try it yourself. See if you can move your skin, or is it tight? Massage your entire head with your fingertips, moving the skin around. Actually move your fingers towards each other and away from each other, as well as round and round, to get the skin to move. Do this for at least 30 seconds to a minute. This massaging might also help to alleviate stress headaches. It helped me, so I hope it will help you.

B. Set up specific time segments for all actions.

I was up at 5:30 a.m. to get kids dressed, lunches ready, and out the door on time. At 7:30 a.m., Mom went to the shop to answer phones and I went to the hospital to see Gary. At about 11 a.m., I went to the shop and let Mom go see Gary for his lunch time. At

2:30 p.m., Mom came back to the shop until her closing time, and I went home to stay with the kids until she came home. I got ready for work and started dinner. She fed, bathed, and tucked the kids into bed as I worked. Going to bed about midnight or 1 a.m., I got about 4, maybe 5, hours of sleep each night that I know of. It usually felt like less. This went on for more than just the long stay at the hospital. It became a routine, and we did not have to think too long on anything.

One thing that Dr. Yee told me was to go to bed at midnight whether I would go to sleep or not. People need at least 4 to 5 hours of sleep within a 24-hour period to be fully functional. At some point, you will get rest and find yourself waking up by the alarm at your regular time. Often, I was awake a few minutes before the alarm went off, but I must have slept for a little while. That was why I did my exercises, so that I would wear myself out before going to bed.

If you find that you don't seem to get any rest, put yourself to bed at least by midnight.

Whether you sleep or not, or even if you find yourself awake a few hours later, your body needs the rest to cope with being required to perform all the caregiver's tasks. Your job is to be functional, even if your loved one cannot.

C. Take an extra five minutes for yourself.

Driving to and from work, driving to a pharmacy by yourself, or getting groceries at the store, these are the times that the caregiver can sneak a couple of minutes to sit and do nothing. I cried and prayed as I sat in the car by the side of the road or parked at a store. It was better to be parked away from most of the people coming in or out of the store, as some got concerned and tapped on my window to ask if I was all right. It's just safer to not be driving and crying at the same time. And I kept a box of tissues in the car for blowing my nose and wiping my face.

If you end up doing this, take a couple of minutes to breathe slowly and calm yourself before driving again. Blink your eyes, pat you face, get the regular color back to your cheeks, and breathe slowly. You don't have to do anything for a minute or two. It's just to have a little peace and quiet for yourself.

D. Giving yourself a break.

After several months of caring for my husband, there were times when I needed to rejuvenate myself, not just take care of keeping Gary's spirits up. We got "cabin fever." We went on vacation even when Gary was feeling the after-effects of the Chemo. It was good to get away from the normal four walls of the home.

About a year after my father began taking care of my mother, he was invited by his old coworkers to go on a weekend, overnight Las Vegas trip. He arranged for Mom to be with a friend who happened to be a nurse. Rather than go by bus, he drove to Las Vegas by himself a day early. He arrived at about 11 or 11:30 p.m. and checked into the hotel. He woke up at about 11 or 11:30 a.m. the next day because he had to go to the bathroom. Dad said he hadn't slept like that the entire year. When he returned, I asked if he felt a little more relaxed and not as tense. Yeah, he did. I also asked him if he felt like he had a little more patience with Mom. Yeah, he did.

Three or four years later with Mom now in a nursing facility, my father had a trip planned to see Holland one last time. It was with a touring group to see not only my mother's relatives in her homeland, but also taking a train ride to see other parts of Europe. It was getting closer and closer for him to fly, but I felt he was feeling guilty about leaving my mother in the facility. We were on vacation as well, and I called him the day before his flight was scheduled. I told him to make sure he got on that plane. He said he didn't think Mom should have to be alone at the nursing facility. I told him she was not alone at all. She was with nurses, a doctor, and other patients, so he did not need to be there. Dad finally admitted he was feeling guilty. I told him he could feel guilty as much as he wanted, but to get his butt on the plane the next day. What finally convinced him was that this might be the last time to see his aging relatives and friends that may not be coming to see him in America.

The body of the caregiver can only take so much abuse. After a year or so, there has to be a break somewhere.

Taking a weekend off really helps to rest the mind and body. But when taking a vacation, the problem may be that the body feels it can relax and take on a cold or flu. This leaves the caregiver very weak and un-rested, quite the opposite of what was planned. I have learned that when I do plan to slip away, I have to be careful just as if I am at home, keeping up my vitamins and exercising just like a regular day. Try not to slack off just because you may get to go on a vacation. Keep up your body's needs so it can go back to work when you get back on the job of care giving.

E. Support for you.

As I cared for Gary, a few people involved kept in contact. My mother-in-law was worried about her son. She depended on me to take care of Gary and the finances. In turn, I depended on her to watch over my boys in the early night while I was at work. My father-in-law, because they were divorced, called several times a month to see if Gary would be alright. He depended on me to care for Gary as well. People at work were supportive of my efforts and gave me sympathy, but they also knew I was the one that had to take care of Gary. My own parents lived too far away to be of help, but they also called several times to see how we were holding up. All these people were helpful on the surface, but there were very few that knew how much deeper the worry and fear was inside me.

Gary's cousins became my support as they lived close enough to us, just to talk to about what was going on. To complain to about being called any number of names but my name. To relax the face front that I managed to keep on when dealing with all the other people. At one point, when Gary's cousin gave my shoulders a hug and squeeze, my knees almost buckled. Here I had been constantly holding up Gary, so it felt strange for someone else to give me a hug that was meant to hold me up. I had to be careful that someone else did not let me break down too much or I would be a wreck for another hour.

These same cousins ended up taking care of their father who became bed-ridden, terminally ill with prostate cancer. I became their support person. They would come over on a moment's notice, waving their arms and telling me about the things the father would say or do just to get a rise out of them. I was able to let them pour out their frustration of loving and hating their father. It was maddening that he did this to them, and as the cousin put it, "He was an ornery cuss until the day he died."

It does not matter how many people help the caregiver: doing errands that need to be done, babysitting kids when needed while you have a sudden trip to the hospital with the ill person, or doing things around the house that needed to be done while you were gone.

Your best support person is the true friend that lets you talk freely about what feelings you, the caregiver, are going through.

The one who gives you the chance to voice out your frustrations. Yes, and maybe cry for a while on their shoulder. You only need one person for this kind of support, so don't feel bad if you can't tell all your friends what is truly going on inside you.

F. Let yourself laugh whenever possible.

The day of Gary's first exploratory surgery was cutting him from stem to stern—that is, from pelvis to sternum—that left him in the hospital room to wake up with me and his mother by his side. Mom did not know what to reply to his first question, "Well, did they get it out?" I answered in like angry voice that "No, they couldn't get it out without letting it into your bloodstream." You can imagine his angry exclamations of frustration.

A while later, his cousin-in-law came to visit to see how he did. Both she, with having had stomach surgery, Mom with having had a hysterectomy, and I with having had two Cesarean Section births, knew what Gary would be facing. The infamous request by the nurse that evening: "Do a cough for me." A small pillow was next to Gary on the bed. We all told him to hold it on his stomach, with staples now in a long row down his front, and then give a small cough to test how much he could do. Yeah, yeah, sure. As the nurse helped him to sit up before going to the chair so she could change the bed sheets, she asked him to cough. Gary had one hand loosely on the pillow, inhaled a breath and coughed like a regular cough.

"OOOOOH!" he cried out as he hugged the little pillow with both hands. Still on the bed, he fell sideways holding the pillow tightly, moaning in pain. All us girls laughed and told him he should have listened to us. We've been through it, and we know what it's like. And we know it hurts.

About six months into the Chemotherapy, it was fine to go out to a restaurant once in a while. Gary was not recognized as the man someone might have known. Just another patron going out to eat. In fact, we risked going on a Thanksgiving vacation at our timeshare unit in Indio, CA. As we dressed nicely for dinner, Gary came out of the bathroom and stood in front of the dresser mirror, looking at his regular, baggy-looking clothes.

"It looks a little loose, huh?" he said as he looked at his image. His shirt was tucked into the pants, zippered up, and belt comfortably on his waist. As he tugged slightly at the pocket to smooth it out, his pants fell down around his knees and ankles. I couldn't help but snicker in laughter.

"That's not funny, Honey, but that *is* funny." We laughed while Gary pulled up his pants again and tucked in his shirt.

"Guess I'll have to be careful about that." He pulled the belt in another notch to tighten it a bit more.

When my mother was admitted to a secured facility where she could walk around without supervision if she wanted to, Dad always made sure she was dressed for the weather. Once, as a windy day called for a sweater, Dad was trying to hold onto her arm to get it on one shoulder. Curious what he was doing, she was turning to him. I was trying to get her other arm in the sleeve as I followed her little circle to get the hole by her hand. Dad was trying to keep the shoulder of the sweater from falling off so I could do that, turning the way she was going. Here, the three of us are turning in a circle as Mom kept looking the other way and I could not get her hand into the hole of the sweater. Around and around we went, laughing as we tried to stop her and get her in. Dad finally had to grab her shoulders to stop her moving. I finally got her hand into the armhole, and we could button her up.

There are moments when something just slightly ridiculous is said or happens that will give you and your loved one a small "comic relief" of the whole situation. Take that moment to laugh or you will go crazy. It helps not only the ill person, it helps you. The old cliché is that "laughter is the best medicine." It gives your heart a lightness that is needed, it relieves some of the pressure of a situation, and it shows that you still love and can laugh with that ill person.

Don't feel bad if something only happens to your loved one. Just apologize while laughing and give them a hug.

Tell them you love them, but *that* (situation/action) was funny.

Chapter 7 – The Survival
A. Physical and mental after-effects.

Now that the actual Chemotherapy was finished, Gary had to have a blood test every month for a year, then every 6 months, and then every year. Now, finally, he does it whenever he has a physical done. After five years, he was declared a Survivor. We get Christmas cards from Dr. Yee, and she later became the Oncology Director for Inter-Community Hospital is Covina, CA.

Physically, Gary grew back his hair, itching in the beginning. Surprisingly, the hair on his head came in straighter than it was before, and darker. Where the curls would get tightly wound by the ends, now were so straight as to stick up until it grew long enough to hair gel it to a side or back. He started out with dark brown hair, but now it was almost black. He was supposed to be my 40-year-old silver-haired fox, like his father. Now I would have to wait another 20 years for it to go white with age. He gained his weight back in a year very slowly, and he did fit into his clothes again.

Gary has trained his lungs to expand better to breathe. He still cannot run without breathing very hard when not getting enough oxygen. At one point, while choosing music in a juke box which was near the bar's door, a man was outside while smoking his cigarette. The smoke was drifting back inside at Gary. After a couple of minutes, he swayed and almost fell off the stool. A friend caught his arm and asked if he felt all right because his face was kind of gray. Gary did not know what happened. Then he smelled the smoke and said he had to move to get air. The second-hand smoke deprived him of oxygen and made him feint.

Now when people smoke near him, he asks them if they will put out the cigarette while he is there. Some smokers are offended, and some will put out the cigarette. If not, he has to move to get away from it. Dr. Yee told Gary that he had to walk to keep his lungs as well as his body exercised. He can walk for miles without any problem and loves to walk the swap meet each weekend.

Fingertips and toes are still numb, and Gary has to wear gloves in cold weather and closed shoes to be safe from injuries. He also still is very hard of hearing because the hairs inside the ears were also destroyed by the Chemotherapy. Tinnitus is a constant companion, and I am constantly repeating what he did not hear from other people or movies in a conversation. A hearing aid was tried, but it not only amplifies the sounds he wants to hear, but it also amplifies the Tinnitus. He has to take a break from wearing a hearing aid for a while to quiet the noise of the Tinnitus.

Gary ended up with another surgery for his intestines. The large intestine got twisted with scar tissue from where the tumor had pushed and injured it. The joke was asking the doctors if they had put in a zipper. He expects he will have another surgery later in his life. He did get left with many surgical clips inside his body and set offs the metal detectors at airports every time. He later had another surgery because of scar tissue, of which two and a half pounds were removed from his abdomen.

Our sons were very grateful that they had a father to grow up with. Dad was able to watch each go through and graduate from high school, and one graduate from the Navy boot camp. I am grateful that he was able to be there to help raise them.

Gary still owns his own business and warehouse. It was physically demanding for a while. Friends of the business came to help get jobs finished that needed to be done. As he gained his strength back, the physical labor became easier, but now he must take breaks to be able to breathe properly. As the owner of the business, he has the advantage that he can take as many breaks as he feels he needs.

As the loved one begins the long journey of healing, if he/she is so lucky to live, many physical changes may have taken place. Disability, whether physical or mental, is evaluated every two years.

If the house you are living in does not help with the body changes, you have to get changes done to the house to make it more accommodating.

If he/she can drive again, make sure their depth perception is up to par again. If the job they do is no longer able to be done, a change of occupancy may have to be learned. For a physically tough job, one might have to learn a desk job to replace a steady income. In other words, a disability need not be permanent. It's just that you may have to help the loved one to learn something else to replace what they used to do.

B. Financial status.

If nothing else, learning to live on a budget was forced into our lives. With budgeting, the bills from the hospital took us five years to get paid off. It may be that you will also need to stay on a budget for all the bills that come after a major illness. Money must be monitored by at least one person in the family, and the caregiver is normally that person. As the healing years begin, having the entire family on board with being careful with money, your lives can still be very happy ones.

After the cancer, Gary and I began taking our vacations very seriously, making sure we budgeted for time off from our daily lives. It still took both of our incomes to live in a nice house, to each have a car to drive, and to take vacations.

Be careful to watch that your budget also includes putting something away in the savings. Outside of that, it may mean that only a night out to a nice dinner is affordable. It may mean that a couple years of not going on vacation will allow a nice trip later.

Calculate what kind of payment your budget can handle if you need to purchase something major, like a washer, a dryer, a stove, a refrigerator, or even a car.

As has happened to us, a major breakdown of our refrigerator had us buying a new one during the first year of Chemotherapy. A discontinued year of a new fridge gave us 50% off the price. A dryer went out and a new one had to be bought in the third year. Even though these were bought on credit, it is the payments that the budget must handle.

C. You and your loved one.

Psychologically, Gary did not notice the world around him more than the length of his arms for a year or more. It was as he began to feel better with actually having a light at the end of that proverbial tunnel that he was noticing everyone else, and especially me. He was still very weak and unstable, but he was not in constant pain anymore. He was noticing the dark circles under my eyes, the look that I was very tired, and that I was very quiet most of the time. I never wanted to argue to keep the peace in the home for all living there. I doggedly went to work each day for fear of losing my job and, therefore, losing my health coverage. I was relying on the health coverage to keep paying for the bills. It felt strange not to have to go to the hospital for days at a time. No more chemicals were needed. No more blood tests, except for once a month. The Hickman catheter for the needles was removed.

My mother-in-law offered to babysit the kids so we could go on a little weekend vacation. We booked a room at a small hotel in Solvang, CA, to relax and enjoy the quaint little town. Traffic was very busy on the freeway, and it took us three hours to get there. We used this time to talk about how things were going, how the kids were holding up, and how his mom had held up her part of the business to answer phones. She brought information to Gary to do the quotes. Then he asked me how I was doing and was there anything that he could do to help, now that he was feeling better.

This was very hard for me. I had been feeling overwhelmed with all the things I was doing. There was one thing that I could now ask of Gary. I asked him to not lean down so hard on me when he gave me a hug. Yes, I know he was easily tired by doing walks or any kind of work, but I was exhausted and was barely standing on my own two feet, let alone try to hold him up anymore. Gary was so sorry that he did that, hadn't realized that he leaned on me when giving me a hug, and promised he would try not to do that anymore. We were both crying at this point. It was just one thing to ask of him now that he was on the road to recovery, but it was a start to help me.

When we got to Solvang and visited a gift store, the man offered to clean and straighten our wedding rings. Both our rings of 14kt gold needed it, but Gary was having a hard time taking off his ring. It was bent into his finger. He had to pull it out with the man's little tool so he could get it off. Wondering how that had happened, Gary figured he had been gripping the steering wheel so hard it had bent his ring almost square.

As the patient begins to recover, should he/she be so

fortunate, the world once again is noticed.

All the overwhelming feelings and tiresome activity of the caregiver will now be noticed by your loved one. There are many things that you would love to ask of him/her to do or not do, but you must be careful. Is what you are going to ask of them something that they actually can do? Try not to ask them to fix the roof, or finish doing the backyard sprinkler system, or start cleaning the whole house again. You know that would be ridiculous and they would not be able to do it physically. But you can ask them to do something simple and small that does not take much effort. Have them fold laundry with you, or wipe some of the car as you both wash it, or even help change the bed sheets.

Take these opportunities to talk about how the kids are growing up so fast, that the car's oil should be changed at an auto shop, and that the next set of sheets you want to be a different color and what does he/she think? It's the small talk that makes the conversation more intimate and personal. It involves them with future images of kids or grandkids graduating from school; that the car does not have to be done by them if not needed; that they have a say in what they want for future bed sheet buying. (Hopefully, the guys don't really care what color bed sheets are.) As the loved one gets stronger, more responsibility of tasks can be taken over again. As long as you begin talking with your loved one again, love will return to a more normal level. The more serious talks can begin as the loved one can handle more and more.

Several people ask me how I can be so patient with my husband. Whenever he is argumentative, ornery, or downright obnoxious, I think about if he had NOT survived, he would not be here at all. I am grateful that he *is* here to be this way, as well as the good person I normally have by my side. Sure, we argue sometimes, but I also found that I cannot be fearful and grateful at the same time.

It may be that if you have a surviving loved one, and as the caregiver, you will need to remember that: You cannot be fearful and grateful at the same time.

Every time the fear looms in your mind, replace it with being grateful that your loved one has survived. But if there seems to be the surety that your loved one will NOT survive, think about the influence that person has had on your life. What was taught to you by a child, a spouse, a parent, a relative, or even a best friend, will live on within your heart, mind, and body. That influence will never go away; therefore, it will live forever within you, even if he/she does pass away. It may help to ease the pain of losing that loved one.

I thank the Good Lord that Gary has survived, that he was there to help raise the boys, that he is physically able to do many things he did before the cancer, and that he is mentally alive and well. He believes God gave him a second chance and he does not want to screw things up (expletive intentionally replaced).

D. You and your family.

As I said before, we now take our vacations very seriously. We still want to travel to different places, experience sights and sounds of theater and music, and write our fantasy books. While the kids were growing up, they also got to travel to a few places, go to theater shows, and still had their dad to cheer them on in school. Gary got to see them both graduate high school, both get the cars of their dreams (one a '64 ½ Ford Mustang, the other a '68 Chevy Rally Sport Camaro), and our youngest graduate from Navy Boot Camp and serve eight years. Now, both boys are married and there are two granddaughters.

The life achievements have been reached, and now we look forward to a retirement future that includes rest and relaxation, a perpetual vacation all the time. We have in mind to write fantasy fiction books, go on cruises, play pool at a local bar, travel around the USA, travel to Europe to see what there is to see, and see a concert/play or two each month. Gary has survived. If nothing else, I feel like I have survived as a caregiver.

If you are lucky enough to still have your loved one, don't think that you will always be in debt with nothing to gain. It is a slow and steady process, and you can't hurry it up any faster. It still seems that time can go by so slowly or it goes by very fast.

Once a year, look at what has been accomplished and plan what will be done for the next year.

It gives you and your loved one a goal to achieve. As your loved one recovers, let the family join in getting things done. Assign duties that they can do for their dad or mom. Let them know that the reward will be for a vacation they can enjoy, even if it is just camping in the summertime. And always tell them you love them.

I hope this will let you know that, as a caregiver, you are not alone in the world, even though it sometimes feels like it. Keeping everything secret does not do you any good for yourself. I hope you have a good friend that you can rely on to hear out your fear, anger, and frustrations for as long as you need. If you strongly need someone to talk to, ask the doctor if they can recommend either a support group in your area or a psychologist. Don't go crazy all by yourself. Join others that have the same feelings and can give you tips to handle different situations. Just remember, you are not alone.

One web site that I had joined on Facebook: **Caregivers Support Group.** They are solely for Caregivers that need to talk to others in the same situation. Or not to talk but to see that others may have some answers to questions you may have. They can give you a lift for you spirit.

May God bless you, the Caregiver.
In Jesus' name, Amen.

P.S.

Do you have any questions? Any other issues you would like to add or should be discussed? Please email me at isabellawalbourne@yahoo.com and let me know. If you enjoyed this booklet, please leave a review in my email as well. Thank you.

www.ingramcontent.com/pod-product-compliance
Lightning Source LLC
Chambersburg PA
CBHW061540050726
47593CB00002B/846